This book was compiled by Daniel Melehi
with the A.I assistance of Inventabot

<u>Dedication</u>

I hope this helps all of my wonderful
readers achieve all their goals in their
business. And I would like to thank my
wonderful wife for all of her continued
support in all my ventures.

©Daniel Melehi

May 7 2023

Contents

Chapter 1: Understanding the Basics of Autoimmune Diseases

Autoimmune diseases are a group of disorders that occur when the immune system mistakenly attacks healthy tissues in the body, resulting in inflammation and tissue damage. There are over 80 different types of autoimmune diseases, each affecting different parts of the body. In this chapter, we'll explore what autoimmune diseases are, how the immune system works, and what causes autoimmune diseases.

SUBCHAPTER 1.1: DEFINING AUTOIMMUNE DISEASES

Autoimmune diseases occur when the immune system, which is designed to protect the body from harmful pathogens such as viruses and bacteria, mistakenly targets healthy cells and tissues in the body. This results in chronic inflammation, which over time can lead to tissue damage and organ failure. The symptoms of autoimmune diseases can vary depending on which part of the body is affected. For example, rheumatoid arthritis primarily affects the joints, while multiple sclerosis affects the central nervous system. Some of the most common symptoms of autoimmune diseases include fatigue, joint pain, skin rashes, and digestive issues.

SUBCHAPTER 1.2: OVERVIEW OF IMMUNE SYSTEM FUNCTION

To understand autoimmune diseases, it's important to have a basic understanding of how the immune system works. The immune system is a complex network of cells, tissues, and organs that work together to defend the body against harmful pathogens. When the immune system encounters a foreign invader, such as a virus or bacterium, it produces antibodies to target and destroy the invader. In autoimmune diseases, the immune system mistakenly targets healthy tissues in the body, producing antibodies that attack those tissues. This can result in chronic inflammation and tissue damage, as the immune system continues to attack healthy cells.

SUBCHAPTER 1.3: CAUSES OF AUTOIMMUNE DISEASES

The exact cause of autoimmune diseases is not fully understood, but several factors have been identified that may contribute to the development of these conditions. These include genetic factors, environmental triggers, and abnormal immune system function. Some autoimmune diseases have a strong genetic component, meaning that they tend to run in families. Environmental triggers, such as infections or exposure to certain drugs or chemicals, may also play a role in triggering the immune system to attack healthy tissues. Abnormal immune system function, such as an overactive immune system or a malfunctioning regulatory system that normally prevents the immune system from attacking healthy tissues, may also contribute to the development of autoimmune diseases. In the next chapter, we'll explore some of the most common myths and misconceptions about autoimmune diseases, including the idea that these conditions are rare or affect only women.

DEFINING AUTOIMMUNE DISEASES

Autoimmune diseases are a group of disorders that occur when the immune system mistakenly attacks healthy cells and tissues in the body. The immune system is designed to protect the body against harmful invaders such as viruses, bacteria, and parasites. However, in individuals with autoimmune diseases, the immune system fails to recognize the difference between healthy cells and foreign invaders, resulting in it attacking healthy tissues and organs. There are over 80 different types of autoimmune diseases, including rheumatoid arthritis, lupus, type 1 diabetes, and multiple sclerosis. These diseases can affect any part of the body and have a wide range of symptoms that can vary from person to person. One unique aspect of autoimmune diseases is that they tend to be chronic, which means they can last for a lifetime. Additionally, autoimmune diseases are usually progressive, meaning they can worsen over time if not properly managed. Unfortunately, the underlying causes of autoimmune diseases are not well understood. However, there are several factors that may contribute to their development, including genetics, environmental factors, and infections. In the next subchapter, we will explore the immune system function in more detail to gain a better understanding of how autoimmune diseases develop.

OVERVIEW OF IMMUNE SYSTEM FUNCTION

The immune system is an intricate network of cells, tissues, and organs that work together to protect the body from harmful pathogens, such as bacteria, viruses, and toxins. Its primary function is to identify and destroy foreign invaders while leaving healthy tissues and cells untouched. The immune system comprises two major components: the innate immune system and the adaptive immune system. The innate immune system is the body's first line of defense against invading pathogens. It includes physical and chemical barriers, as well as immune cells such as neutrophils, monocytes, and natural killer cells. These cells have pre-existing mechanisms that can immediately attack and destroy pathogens. Additionally, they can activate other immune cells to fight off the infection. The adaptive immune system, on the other hand, is more specific and tailored to detect and eliminate specific pathogens. This type of immunity is slower to respond than the innate immune system, but its response time improves with repeat exposures. The adaptive immune system includes T cells and B cells, which work together to produce antibodies, residing in the blood or tissues, that can recognize, bind to, and destroy the specific pathogen. As the immune system fights off infections, it keeps track of the pathogens it has encountered. This allows it to respond more quickly and efficiently to future invasions by the same pathogen. It is important to note that the immune system is not always flawless. Sometimes, it can become overactive and attack healthy tissues and cells, leading to autoimmune diseases. In these cases, the immune system mistakes the body's own tissues and organs as foreign invaders and targets them for destruction. Understanding the mechanisms that drive the immune response is crucial for developing effective treatments for autoimmune diseases.

SUBCHAPTER 1.3: CAUSES OF AUTOIMMUNE DISEASES

Scientists and doctors still do not know the exact causes of autoimmune diseases. They do know that autoimmune diseases are caused by a combination of genetic and environmental factors. Some of the factors that may trigger autoimmune diseases include:

1. Genetics:

Autoimmune diseases tend to cluster in families, which suggests that there is a genetic component to their development. However, having a family member with an autoimmune disease does not necessarily mean that you will develop one too. Researchers have identified specific genes that may increase one's susceptibility to autoimmune diseases.

2. Environmental Factors:

Environmental triggers such as infections or exposure to chemicals, or other toxins are thought to play a significant role in triggering autoimmune diseases. In some cases, autoimmune diseases may be triggered by stress. For example, an individual may have a genetic susceptibility to an autoimmune disease, but it only develops after a viral infection.

3. Gender:

Women are more likely to develop autoimmune diseases than men. Researchers do not know why, but many theories suggest that hormones or genetic factors could be responsible.

4. Age:

Autoimmune diseases can develop at any age but are most commonly diagnosed during childbearing years. Additionally, researchers believe that there is a complex interplay between the immune system and other systems in the body. Dysfunction in one system can lead to dysfunction in another, ultimately causing an autoimmune disease to develop. While we may not be able to prevent autoimmune diseases entirely, by understanding the possible triggers, we may be able to reduce their likelihood by avoiding specific environmental factors that could trigger their development.

Chapter 2: Debunking Myths About Autoimmune Diseases

Autoimmune diseases are often misunderstood, and this chapter will debunk common myths about them. It is important to understand the truth about autoimmune diseases to prevent misinformation.

SUBCHAPTER 2.1: AUTOIMMUNE DISEASES ARE RARE

Contrary to popular belief, autoimmune diseases are not rare. In fact, they are prevalent around the world. According to the American Autoimmune Related Diseases Association, approximately 50 million Americans have autoimmune diseases. This makes them more common than heart disease and cancer. While some autoimmune diseases are less common than others, such as Addison's disease or

Wegener's granulomatosis, many others are widespread, like the ones we will discuss in chapter 3.

Fact:

Autoimmune diseases are not rare. They affect more than 50 million Americans, making them more common than heart disease and cancer.

SUBCHAPTER 2.2: AUTOIMMUNE DISEASES ONLY AFFECT WOMEN

Another common myth is that autoimmune diseases only affect women. While it's true that women are more likely to develop autoimmune diseases, men can also get them. In fact, some autoimmune diseases affect men more than women. Women are more likely to develop autoimmune diseases due to hormonal and genetic differences. However, men can still develop autoimmune diseases, and everyone should be aware of their symptoms.

Fact:

Autoimmune diseases can affect both men and women, although women are more likely to develop them due to hormonal and genetic differences.

SUBCHAPTER 2.3: AUTOIMMUNE DISEASES CANNOT BE TREATED

Finally, some people believe that there are no treatments for autoimmune diseases and that they are incurable. This is not true. While there is no definitive cure for autoimmune diseases, there are a variety of treatments available that can help manage symptoms. Medications like immunosuppressants and steroids can help control inflammation and slow the progression of the disease. Lifestyle changes like exercise and stress reduction can also help manage symptoms. In addition, advancements in research are leading to new treatments that may one day cure autoimmune diseases.

Fact:

While there is no definitive cure for autoimmune diseases, there are treatments available that can help manage symptoms. These include medications, lifestyle changes, and advancements in medical research. In conclusion, understanding the truth about autoimmune diseases is essential. Debunking common myths about these diseases can help people get the right diagnosis and treatment. The next chapter will discuss some of the most common autoimmune diseases in more detail.

SUBCHAPTER 2.1: AUTOIMMUNE DISEASES ARE RARE

Despite the growing awareness about autoimmune diseases, many people still believe that these conditions are rare. In reality, this is far from the truth. Autoimmune diseases are actually quite common and affect millions of people around the world. In fact, autoimmune diseases are more prevalent than heart disease, which is often considered the leading cause of death globally. The statistics are staggering - out of the 50 million Americans suffering from chronic diseases, a whopping 23.5 million suffer from autoimmune diseases. That's nearly one in every 13 people in the US! Another common myth is that autoimmune diseases only affect older people. This is simply not true as autoimmune diseases can affect anyone, regardless of age or gender. While some autoimmune diseases are more common in certain age groups or genders, many can strike anyone at any age. Furthermore, autoimmune diseases can be difficult to diagnose as their symptoms can be similar to other health conditions. This can lead to a delay in diagnosis and treatment, which can worsen the impact on the patient's life. It is important to raise awareness about the prevalence of autoimmune diseases so that people can recognize the symptoms and seek medical attention early on. The earlier the diagnosis, the better the chances of successfully managing the symptoms and preventing long-term damage to the body. In conclusion, autoimmune diseases are not rare. They are a common chronic illness affecting millions of people worldwide, with a wide range of symptoms and diseases that can develop at any age. It is essential to change the misconception that these conditions are rare and to promote awareness so that patients have access to early diagnosis, better treatments, and improved quality of life.

SUBCHAPTER 2.2: AUTOIMMUNE DISEASES ONLY AFFECT WOMEN

It is a common misconception that autoimmune diseases only affect women. In reality, autoimmune diseases can affect anyone, regardless of their gender or age. However, it is true that women are more likely to develop autoimmune diseases than men, and some autoimmune diseases are more common in women. For example, diseases like lupus, multiple sclerosis, and rheumatoid arthritis are more common in women. In fact, women are approximately three times more likely to develop autoimmune diseases than men. The reasons for this are not yet fully understood, but researchers believe that hormonal, genetic, and environmental factors may contribute to the gender disparity. It is important to note that while some autoimmune diseases are more prevalent in women, men are still at risk of developing them. Men who do develop autoimmune diseases may face unique challenges, and their symptoms and treatments may differ from those of women. It is crucial to dispel the misconception that autoimmune diseases only affect women. This stereotype can lead to men not being properly diagnosed or receiving appropriate treatment for their symptoms. Healthcare professionals should be aware of the gender disparity in autoimmune diseases and should not allow gender biases to impact their diagnosis and treatment decisions. In conclusion, autoimmune diseases can affect anyone, regardless of their gender. While women are more likely to develop autoimmune diseases, men are still at risk and should seek medical attention if they experience any symptoms. Healthcare professionals must be aware of the gender disparity and not allow gender biases to impact their diagnosis and treatment decisions.

SUBCHAPTER 2.3: AUTOIMMUNE DISEASES CANNOT BE TREATED

One of the most common misconceptions about autoimmune diseases is that they cannot be treated. This is simply not true. While there is no cure for autoimmune diseases, there are various treatment options that can help manage symptoms and improve quality of life. The goal of treatment is to control the immune response, reduce inflammation, and minimize damage to organs and tissues. The type of treatment prescribed will depend on the specific autoimmune disease and the severity of symptoms. Some of the commonly used treatments include immunosuppressants, corticosteroids, and biologic drugs. Immunosuppressants work by suppressing the activity of the immune system, while corticosteroids reduce inflammation. Biologic drugs target specific molecules in the immune system to block their activity and reduce inflammation. In addition to medications, lifestyle changes can also play a crucial role in managing autoimmune diseases. Eating a balanced diet, getting enough rest, and exercising regularly can help improve overall health and reduce symptoms. It is important to work closely with a healthcare provider to develop a personalized treatment plan for managing autoimmune diseases. With the right treatment, many people with autoimmune diseases are able to lead healthy and fulfilling lives.

Chapter 3: Common Autoimmune Diseases

Autoimmune diseases affect millions of people across the globe, and there are various types of autoimmune diseases that can cause different symptoms and complications. In this chapter, we will discuss some of the most common autoimmune diseases.

SUBCHAPTER 3.1: RHEUMATOID ARTHRITIS

Rheumatoid Arthritis (RA) is a chronic autoimmune disease that affects the joints of the body. RA happens when the immune system mistakenly attacks the body's own tissues causing pain, stiffness, swelling, and joint damage. The symptoms of RA generally start with smaller joints, such as hands and feet, and progressively move to larger joints like knees and shoulders. The disease can be managed with disease-modifying antirheumatic drugs (DMARDs), which help relieve inflammation and slow down joint damage.

SUBCHAPTER 3.2: LUPUS

Lupus is a chronic autoimmune disease that can affect any organ or system in the body. The immune system attacks healthy cells and tissues, causing inflammation, pain, and damage to various body parts such as the skin, joints, kidneys, brain, and blood vessels. Symptoms of lupus can be mild or severe, and they can appear and disappear without warning. There is no cure for lupus, but treatments such as corticosteroids, immunosuppressants, and antimalarial drugs can help manage the symptoms and prevent complications.

SUBCHAPTER 3.3: MULTIPLE SCLEROSIS

Multiple Sclerosis (MS) is a chronic autoimmune disease that affects the central nervous system. In MS, the immune system attacks the protective covering of nerve fibers, known as myelin, resulting in nerve damage and communication problems between the brain and other parts of the body. As a result, people with MS may experience symptoms such as vision problems, muscle weakness, difficulty with coordination, and cognitive impairment. Currently, there is no cure for MS, but disease-modifying therapies such as interferon beta-1a and glatiramer acetate can help manage the symptoms and slow down the progression of the disease. In conclusion, autoimmune diseases are a group of conditions that can affect people of all ages and can cause diverse symptoms. In the next chapter, we will discuss the diagnosis and treatment options available for autoimmune diseases.

SUBCHAPTER 3.1: RHEUMATOID ARTHRITIS

Rheumatoid Arthritis (RA) is an autoimmune disease that primarily affects the joints. It is a chronic condition that causes inflammation, pain, stiffness, and loss of function in the joints. RA can also cause inflammation in other parts of the body, such as the lungs, heart, and eyes. Although the exact cause of RA is still unknown, it is believed to be caused by a combination of genetic and environmental factors. Women are two to three times more likely to develop RA than men, and it can develop at any age. The symptoms of RA can vary from person to person, but the most common symptoms include joint pain, stiffness, swelling, and tenderness. These symptoms can occur on both sides of the body and can be most severe in the morning or after periods of inactivity. RA can also cause fatigue, fever, weight loss, and a general feeling of malaise. Diagnosis of RA involves a combination of physical examination, medical history, and imaging tests. Blood tests may also be used to detect certain antibodies that are associated with RA. Early diagnosis and treatment of RA is essential to prevent joint damage and improve outcomes. Treatment of RA involves a combination of medication, physical therapy, and lifestyle changes. Medications used to treat RA include nonsteroidal anti-inflammatory drugs (NSAIDs), disease-modifying antirheumatic drugs (DMARDs), and biologic agents. Physical therapy can help to improve joint function and mobility, while lifestyle changes such as exercise and maintaining a healthy weight can also be beneficial. Living with RA can be challenging, but there are a variety of resources available to help individuals with the condition. Support groups, educational resources, and assistive devices can all help to improve quality of life for people with RA. In conclusion, Rheumatoid Arthritis is a chronic autoimmune disease that primarily affects the joints. Early diagnosis and treatment are crucial in preventing joint damage and improving outcomes for those with RA. By utilizing a combination of medication, physical therapy, and lifestyle changes, individuals with RA can successfully manage their symptoms and improve their overall wellbeing.

CHAPTER 3: COMMON AUTOIMMUNE DISEASES

Subchapter 3.2: Lupus

Lupus, also known as systemic lupus erythematosus (SLE), is a chronic autoimmune disease that affects various parts of the body, including the skin, joints, kidneys, and other organs. Lupus occurs when the immune system attacks healthy cells and tissues in the body, causing inflammation and tissue damage. One of the most distinctive characteristics of lupus is the butterfly-shaped rash that appears on the cheeks and bridge of the nose. However, not all people with lupus develop this rash. Other common symptoms of lupus include joint pain and stiffness, fatigue, fever, chest pain, and shortness of breath. Lupus affects women more often than men, and it typically develops between the ages of 15 and 44. However, anyone can develop lupus regardless of age or gender. The exact cause of lupus is unknown, but certain factors are thought to contribute to its development, including genetics, hormones, and environmental triggers such as infections or exposure to sunlight. There is no cure for lupus, but the condition can be managed with medications and lifestyle changes. The goals of treatment for lupus are to control inflammation, prevent flare-ups, and protect organs from damage. Common medications used to treat lupus include nonsteroidal anti-inflammatory drugs (NSAIDs), corticosteroids, and disease-modifying antirheumatic drugs (DMARDs). In severe cases, immunosuppressant medications may also be used to suppress the immune system and prevent it from attacking the body's healthy cells and tissues. In addition to medication, people with lupus can also benefit from lifestyle changes such as getting regular exercise, getting enough rest, avoiding triggers such as sunlight and stress, and eating a healthy, balanced diet. If you have lupus, it's important to work closely with your healthcare team to manage your symptoms and prevent complications. With the right treatment and self-care measures, most people with lupus are able to lead active, fulfilling lives.

CHAPTER 3: COMMON AUTOIMMUNE DISEASES

Subchapter 3.3: Multiple Sclerosis

Multiple sclerosis (MS) is a chronic progressive autoimmune disease that affects the myelin sheath that covers the nerve fibers in the spinal cord and brain. MS is a debilitating disease that impairs the communication between the brain and other parts of the body. As an autoimmune disease, multiple sclerosis occurs when the body's immune system mistakenly attacks the protective covering (myelin) that surrounds nerve fibers in your central nervous system. This leads to inflammation and damage to the myelin sheath, which slows down or blocks electrical signals from traveling through the brain and spinal cord to the rest of the body. The symptoms of MS can vary greatly from person to person and may include vision problems, numbness or tingling in limbs, loss of coordination, weakness, fatigue, and cognitive impairment. The cause of multiple sclerosis is still unknown, but it is believed to be a combination of genetic and environmental factors. There is currently no cure for multiple sclerosis, but there are a variety of treatment options available to help manage symptoms and slow the progression of the disease. Medications such as corticosteroids, interferons, and immunosuppressants can be prescribed to help reduce swelling and inflammation in the central nervous system. Physical therapy can also help improve strength, flexibility, and balance. Occupational therapy can help people with MS adapt to changes in their abilities and learn new skills to maintain their independence. In addition, healthy lifestyle modifications like regular exercise and a healthy diet can also play an important role in managing multiple sclerosis symptoms. In recent years, there have been significant advances in MS research, including the development of new medications, diagnostic tests, and improved imaging techniques. Scientists are also working to better understand the underlying causes of the disease, which may eventually lead to a cure. Overall, while multiple sclerosis can be a challenging disease to manage, there are a range of treatment options available to help improve quality of life and slow the progression of the disease. It is important for anyone living with MS to work closely with their healthcare team to develop a comprehensive treatment plan that meets their unique needs.

Chapter 4: Diagnosis and Treatment of Autoimmune Diseases

Autoimmune diseases are challenging to diagnose, but once a diagnosis is made, there are several treatment options available to manage symptoms. In this chapter, we will explore the common diagnostic tests used in diagnosing autoimmune diseases and the various medications and lifestyle changes that can help treat them.

SUBCHAPTER 4.1: COMMON DIAGNOSTIC TESTS

The diagnosis of an autoimmune disease is not always straightforward and requires a combination of medical history, physical examinations, and laboratory testing. The following are some of the common diagnostic tests used to diagnose autoimmune diseases:

Blood Tests

Blood tests are often the first step in diagnosing autoimmune diseases. These tests look for specific antibodies and proteins that are associated with particular autoimmune diseases. For example, a blood test for rheumatoid arthritis looks for the presence of rheumatoid factor (RF) and anti-cyclic citrullinated peptide (anti-CCP) antibodies.

Antinuclear Antibody Test (ANA)

The antinuclear antibody test (ANA) is a blood test that looks for the presence of certain antibodies in the blood that react with nuclear antigens. An elevated ANA level is often an indication of an autoimmune disease, but it is not specific to one disease.

Biopsy

A biopsy involves taking a small sample of tissue from an affected area of the body for examination under a microscope. Biopsies can provide valuable information about the specific type of autoimmune disease affecting an individual.

SUBCHAPTER 4.2: MEDICATIONS USED IN TREATING AUTOIMMUNE DISEASES

Treating rheumatic diseases involves a combination of medication and lifestyle changes. While there is no cure for autoimmune diseases, several medications can help manage symptoms and slow the progression of the disease. The following are some commonly used medications in treating autoimmune diseases:

Nonsteroidal Anti-inflammatory Drugs (NSAIDs)

NSAIDs, such as ibuprofen and aspirin, are commonly used to treat the pain and inflammation associated with autoimmune diseases.

Corticosteroids

Corticosteroids, such as prednisone, are powerful anti-inflammatory drugs that can help manage the symptoms of autoimmune diseases. They are often used in combination with other medications.

Disease-Modifying Anti-Rheumatic Drugs (DMARDs)

DMARDs, such as methotrexate and leflunomide, are drugs that can help slow the progression of autoimmune diseases by suppressing the immune system.

Biologic Agents

Biologic agents, such as etanercept and infliximab, are genetically engineered drugs that block specific components of the immune system that contribute to autoimmune diseases.

SUBCHAPTER 4.3: LIFESTYLE CHANGES FOR MANAGING SYMPTOMS

In addition to medication, lifestyle changes can also be helpful in managing the symptoms of autoimmune diseases. Some lifestyle changes that can help include:

Diet

A healthy diet can help manage inflammation and promote overall health. Anti-inflammatory diets that include plenty of fruits, vegetables, lean proteins, and healthy fats are recommended.

Exercise

Regular exercise can help manage the symptoms of autoimmune diseases by promoting joint mobility and reducing inflammation.

Stress Management

Stress can trigger autoimmune symptoms, so it is essential to manage stress levels. Mind-body practices, such as yoga and meditation, can be helpful in managing stress.

Smoking Cessation

Smoking can exacerbate the symptoms of autoimmune diseases, so smoking cessation is strongly recommended. With a combination of diagnostic tests, medication, and lifestyle changes, it is possible to manage the symptoms of autoimmune diseases and enjoy a good quality of life. In the next chapter, we will explore the challenges associated with coping with autoimmune diseases.

COMMON DIAGNOSTIC TESTS

Diagnosing autoimmune diseases can be tricky as their symptoms are often similar to other medical conditions. However, there are several diagnostic tests that doctors can perform to confirm the presence of an autoimmune disease. **Blood tests:** Blood tests are the most important diagnostic tool for autoimmune diseases. A variety of blood tests can detect the autoimmune response, including tests that look for the presence of specific autoantibodies. For example, the anti-nuclear antibody (ANA) test is used to look for antibodies that target the nuclei of cells. In addition, tests that measure levels of inflammation and markers in the blood can point to the presence of an autoimmune disorder. **Biopsy:** Biopsy is another important diagnostic tool. In some cases, a biopsy of affected tissue may be taken and examined by a pathologist. This can help to confirm the diagnosis and help to determine the best course of treatment. **Imaging tests:** Imaging tests can help doctors to visualize the affected organs and tissues. Common examples of imaging tests used to diagnose autoimmune diseases include MRI and ultrasound. **Physical examination:** During a physical exam, a doctor will look for signs of inflammation and damage to the organs or tissues. This can include joint tenderness or swelling, skin rashes or lesions, or swollen glands. It's important to note that diagnosing an autoimmune disease can be a complex process that often requires the involvement of multiple specialists, including rheumatologists and immunologists. However, with the right diagnostic tests and a thorough examination, doctors can accurately diagnose autoimmune diseases and help patients receive the treatments they need.

SUBCHAPTER 4.2: MEDICATIONS USED IN TREATING AUTOIMMUNE DISEASES

While there's no cure for autoimmune diseases, there are a variety of medications available to help manage symptoms, reduce inflammation, and slow down the progression of the disease. The type of medication prescribed by a doctor will depend on the specific autoimmune disease a patient has, as well as the severity of their symptoms. One of the most commonly prescribed types of medication for autoimmune diseases are anti-inflammatory drugs, such as nonsteroidal anti-inflammatory drugs (NSAIDs), corticosteroids, and disease-modifying antirheumatic drugs (DMARDs). NSAIDs and corticosteroids work by reducing inflammation in the body, which can help to alleviate symptoms like pain and swelling. DMARDs, on the other hand, work by suppressing the immune system, preventing it from attacking healthy tissues. Immunosuppressant drugs are another type of medication that can be prescribed for autoimmune diseases. These drugs work by suppressing the immune system, which can help to reduce inflammation and slow down the progression of the disease. However, because these drugs can increase the risk of infections and other health problems, they are usually only prescribed in severe cases.

Biologic response modifiers are a relatively new type of medication that have been developed specifically for treating autoimmune diseases. These drugs work by targeting specific parts of the immune system, in order to reduce inflammation and prevent the immune system from attacking healthy tissues. While these medications can be highly effective, they are also quite expensive and may not be covered by insurance. Finally, there are certain types of medications that are used to manage specific symptoms of autoimmune diseases. For example, some patients may be prescribed muscle relaxants or painkillers to manage muscle spasms or chronic pain. Others may be prescribed medications that help to improve overall mental health and wellbeing, such as antidepressants or anti-anxiety medications. It's important to note that while medications can be highly effective in managing symptoms of autoimmune diseases, they can also come with a variety of side effects. Patients should always talk to their doctor about any potential risks and benefits associated with a medication before starting a new treatment plan. Additionally, it's important to be diligent about taking medications as prescribed and to attend all scheduled doctor appointments to ensure that the treatment plan is working effectively.

SUBCHAPTER 4.3: LIFESTYLE CHANGES FOR MANAGING SYMPTOMS

While medications can be effective in treating autoimmune diseases, making certain lifestyle changes can also help manage symptoms and improve quality of life. Here are some lifestyle changes that may help:

Diet Modifications

Research has shown that certain foods can trigger inflammation, and it is recommended that those with autoimmune diseases avoid or limit their consumption.

For instance, foods such as gluten, dairy, sugar, processed foods, and fried foods have been known for triggering inflammation in some patients. On the other hand, adding anti-inflammatory foods like leafy greens, fatty fish, fruits, and vegetables to one's diet can help reduce inflammation. Incorporating low-carbohydrate and high-fat content diets like keto and paleo has proved to be beneficial for some people with autoimmune disorders.

Exercise

Regular physical activity can help improve overall immune system function and mood. However, it is essential to find the right balance of exercise as excessive physical activity can worsen symptoms. Engaging in low-impact activities like yoga, swimming, and cycling can help improve muscle strength and flexibility without causing flare-ups.

Stress Management

Chronic stress can lead to inflammation and exacerbate autoimmune symptoms. Engaging in stress management activities like deep breathing, meditation, and relaxation techniques can help reduce stress levels. Joining support groups, working with a therapist, and practicing self-care regularly can also help manage stress and improve overall well-being.

Sleep Quality

Sleep is crucial for the body to repair itself, and those with autoimmune diseases may need more sleep than others. Proper sleep hygiene is essential, making adjustments like having a regular sleep and wake time, limiting exposure to electronics before bedtime and creating a comfortable sleep environment with the right kind of bedding and lighting. These measures can help manage fatigue, a prevalent symptom in patients suffering from autoimmune disorders. These are just a few lifestyle changes that can help manage the symptoms of autoimmune diseases. It's worth keeping an open mind and trying out different methods as each person's body responds differently. It's important to note that creating an individualized plan with a doctor and other health professionals is crucial for managing symptoms and preventing disease progression.

Chapter 5: Coping with Autoimmune Diseases

Living with an autoimmune disease can be a challenging and frustrating experience. Coping with the physical symptoms, emotional issues, and lifestyle adjustments can be overwhelming. However, with the right coping strategies, it is possible to lead a full and meaningful life. In this chapter, we will explore the various coping mechanisms that can help individuals with autoimmune diseases manage their condition and maintain their quality of life.

SUBCHAPTER 5.1: MENTAL HEALTH CHALLENGES ASSOCIATED WITH AUTOIMMUNE DISEASES

Living with an autoimmune disease can have a significant impact on one's mental health. Coping with chronic pain, fatigue, and other physical symptoms can lead to depression, anxiety, and other mental health challenges. It is important for individuals with autoimmune diseases to recognize and address these issues to maintain their overall well-being. One way to manage mental health challenges is through therapy or counseling. A therapist can help individuals develop coping mechanisms and strategies to manage their emotional responses to their disease. Support groups can also be beneficial, as they offer a platform for individuals to connect and support one another.

SUBCHAPTER 5.2: SUPPORT GROUPS AND RESOURCES FOR PEOPLE WITH AUTOIMMUNE DISEASES

Support groups can be a valuable resource for individuals with autoimmune diseases. They offer a platform for individuals to connect with others who can relate to their experiences and provide emotional support. Many support groups also provide educational resources and practical advice for managing the disease. In addition to support groups, there are also several online resources available for individuals with autoimmune diseases. Websites and online communities offer a wealth of information and resources for managing the disease, connecting with others, and accessing information about treatment options and clinical trials.

SUBCHAPTER 5.3: TIPS FOR COPING WITH AUTOIMMUNE DISEASES

In addition to therapy, counseling, and support groups, there are several coping mechanisms that individuals with autoimmune diseases can use to manage their condition. Some tips include: - Prioritizing self-care, such as practicing relaxation techniques, getting adequate sleep, and eating a healthy diet - Staying active with low-impact exercises, such as yoga or swimming - Communicating effectively with healthcare providers and advocating for one's own healthcare needs - Finding ways to reduce stress, such as practicing meditation or taking up a creative hobby By incorporating these coping mechanisms into one's daily routine, it is possible to manage the physical and emotional challenges of living with an autoimmune disease and lead a fulfilling life.

CONCLUSION

Living with an autoimmune disease requires patience, resilience, and the right tools for coping. By seeking support from therapy or counseling, joining a support group, and implementing healthy habits, individuals with autoimmune diseases can learn to manage their symptoms and maintain a sense of control over their lives. In the next chapter, we will explore the future of autoimmune disease research and potential cures for these conditions.

SUBCHAPTER 5.1: MENTAL HEALTH CHALLENGES ASSOCIATED WITH AUTOIMMUNE DISEASES

Living with an autoimmune disease can be challenging on different levels, one of which is the impact it has on mental health. Many individuals with autoimmune diseases often experience a range of mental health issues that can affect their quality of life. One of the major mental health challenges associated with autoimmune diseases is depression. Studies have shown that those with autoimmune diseases, especially women, are more likely to experience depression than people without these conditions. This can occur for various reasons, including fatigue, pain, and the fact that living with a chronic illness can be frustrating and tiring. It is crucial to address depression in individuals with autoimmune diseases so that they can receive appropriate treatment and support. Another mental health issue that is strongly associated with autoimmune diseases is anxiety. Those with autoimmune diseases often experience anxiety due to the fear of unpredictable flare-ups, which may cause a significant impact on daily life. Social anxiety and panic attacks are also common among people living with autoimmune diseases as they may fear being judged for their disabilities and how they look. Lastly, autoimmune diseases can also impact an individual's cognitive function, causing difficulties with thinking, concentration, memory, and decision-making. Brain fog, which is a term used to describe issues with memory and concentration, is a common symptom among those with autoimmune diseases. This can cause frustration for those affected as it can negatively affect their daily performance, their ability to work, and even their personal relationships. It is important to acknowledge that mental health challenges are prevalent among individuals living with autoimmune diseases. If you are struggling with your mental health, seek support from a mental health professional or a support group. You are not alone, and there is no shame in seeking help.

SUPPORT GROUPS AND RESOURCES FOR PEOPLE WITH AUTOIMMUNE DISEASES

A diagnosis of autoimmune disease can be overwhelming, leaving people feeling isolated and alone. However, it is essential to understand that you are not alone. There are a variety of resources available that can provide the help, information, and support you need to manage your condition effectively. One essential resource for people with autoimmune diseases is support groups. Support groups can be an excellent source of information on your condition, and they can also provide you with emotional support and encouragement. By sharing their experiences and insights, others dealing with an autoimmune disease can help you develop coping strategies for dealing with the physical and mental challenges that often come with these conditions. There are numerous support groups available that cater to the needs of people with autoimmune diseases. Some of these groups are condition-specific, such as those for lupus or rheumatoid arthritis, while others are more general, focusing on autoimmune diseases as a whole. In addition to support groups, there are many resources available online that can provide valuable information and support. Many non-profit organizations offer information on their websites regarding various autoimmune diseases, as well as forums and chat rooms where people can connect with others dealing with similar challenges. Another essential resource is healthcare providers, including rheumatologists, dermatologists, and other specialists trained in treating autoimmune diseases. These professionals can provide you with information about available treatments, lifestyle changes that may improve your condition, and resources for coping with your emotions and managing stress. Finally, it is important to maintain open communication with family and friends regarding your condition. Educating loved ones about your illness can help build understanding and foster a supportive environment. In conclusion, support groups and resources for people with autoimmune diseases play a crucial role in providing the help, information, and support people need to manage these complex conditions effectively. By connecting with others who are dealing with similar challenges, accessing online resources, and working closely with healthcare providers, people with autoimmune diseases can gain the skills and support needed to live healthy, fulfilling lives.

SUBCHAPTER 5.3: TIPS FOR COPING WITH AUTOIMMUNE DISEASES

Coping with autoimmune diseases can be a challenging experience. Managing chronic symptoms, dealing with flare-ups, and juggling medications and doctor appointments can take a toll on a person's daily life. However, there are several tips and techniques that can help individuals with autoimmune diseases to manage their condition and improve their quality of life. First and foremost, it is vital to prioritize self-care. This includes getting sufficient rest, eating a healthy diet, and engaging in regular exercise. It is natural for individuals with autoimmune diseases to feel fatigued or experience pain, but gentle exercise, such as yoga or tai chi, can help to reduce symptoms and improve mental health. Additionally, developing a routine sleeping schedule and avoiding stressors can help to reduce flare-ups. Another valuable tip for coping with autoimmune diseases is to seek out support groups. Being part of a community of people who share similar experiences can be incredibly validating and help alleviate feelings of loneliness and isolation. Support groups can also be a great source of advice, information, and empathy. Online forums can also be particularly useful for individuals who are too ill to attend in-person meetings. It is also important for individuals to learn as much as possible about their condition. This includes understanding how the disease affects the body, what medications and treatments are available, and what lifestyle changes can make a positive impact. Keeping informed can help individuals to take an active role in their healthcare and improve their overall well-being. Lastly, seeking professional help is crucial for individuals struggling to cope with autoimmune diseases. In addition to medical professionals, therapists and counselors can provide emotional support, coping strategies, and stress management techniques. Medication, meditation, and cognitive-behavioral therapy are also effective treatments for anxiety and depression, which can often be exacerbated by autoimmune diseases. In conclusion, managing autoimmune diseases can be difficult, but there are several ways to cope with the condition and improve quality of life. Prioritizing self-care, seeking out support groups, educating oneself, and seeking professional help are all crucial steps that can help individuals to better manage their condition and live fulfilling lives.

Chapter 6: The Future of Autoimmune Disease Research

Autoimmune diseases affect millions of people worldwide, and while there has been significant progress made in the field of autoimmune disease research, much work remains to be done. In this chapter, we will discuss the future of autoimmune disease research and what promising areas researchers are exploring in their quest to better understand and ultimately cure these complex diseases.

SUBCHAPTER 6.1: PROMISING AREAS OF RESEARCH

One of the most promising areas of autoimmune disease research involves exploring the gut microbiome's role in disease development. The microbiome, which consists of trillions of bacteria living in our gut, plays an essential role in immune system function. Researchers are investigating how changes in the gut microbiome could contribute to the development or progression of autoimmune diseases and identifying strategies to manipulate the microbiome to improve immune function. Another exciting area of research is the use of gene editing technologies such as CRISPR to treat or even cure autoimmune diseases. Scientists are exploring ways to use gene editing to target and modify genes that are involved in the development of autoimmune diseases, as well as ways to modify immune cells to reduce the abnormal response seen in autoimmune diseases. Finally, researchers are exploring the role of environmental factors in the development of autoimmune diseases. Exposure to toxins, pollutants, and infections can all contribute to the development of autoimmunity, and scientists are investigating how these factors interact with the immune system and contribute to disease development.

SUBCHAPTER 6.2: POTENTIAL CURES FOR AUTOIMMUNE DISEASES

While there is still much to learn about autoimmune diseases, several potential cures are being investigated. One of the most promising approaches is the use of immune system modulation therapies. These therapies aim to restore normal immune function and prevent the immune system from attacking the body's tissues. Scientists are also exploring the use of regenerative medicine to repair tissues damaged by autoimmune diseases. In addition, researchers are exploring ways to prevent autoimmune diseases through early intervention. Identifying individuals at high risk for developing autoimmune diseases and providing preventive therapies could significantly reduce the burden of these diseases on individuals and society.

SUBCHAPTER 6.3: COLLABORATIONS IN AUTOIMMUNE DISEASE RESEARCH

Collaboration among researchers, healthcare providers, and patients is critical for advancing autoimmune disease research. For example, online patient communities provide researchers with valuable data about disease symptoms, progression, and treatment outcomes. Patients can also participate in clinical trials to help researchers understand the effectiveness of new therapies and treatment approaches. Healthcare providers play a critical role in autoimmune disease research by providing data and insights into disease patterns and patient outcomes. Researchers can also collaborate with industry partners to develop new therapies and bring them to market.

CONCLUSION

While autoimmune diseases are complex and challenging to understand, significant progress has been made in the field of autoimmune disease research. By continuing to explore promising areas of research, identifying potential cures, and collaborating with patients, healthcare providers, and industry partners, researchers can improve our understanding of autoimmune diseases and develop new and effective treatments that benefit patients worldwide.

SUBCHAPTER 6.1: PROMISING AREAS OF RESEARCH

Autoimmune diseases have long been a mystery to medical professionals. Nevertheless, with recent advancements in medical technology, new discoveries have come to light, offering hope for the future. Here are some areas of research that show promise for the future of autoimmune disease treatment:

1. Genetics Research

Thanks to the Human Genome Project, researchers have identified various genes that may be responsible for triggering autoimmune diseases. Scientists are working to uncover more information about how these genes work and how they can be modified to prevent or lessen the severity of autoimmune diseases.

2. Immune System Cell Research

Scientists are investigating how immune system cells interact with each other and how they function in those with autoimmune diseases. They hope to find new ways to identify which cells are causing problems and how to deactivate them.

3. Gut Health and Microbiome Research

Researchers are studying the connection between gut health and autoimmune diseases. They believe that the microbiome (the bacteria that live in your gut) may also play a significant role in autoimmune diseases. Studies have shown that changes in the microbiome may influence the development or severity of autoimmune diseases.

4. Stem Cell Research

Stem cell therapy is gaining popularity as a potential treatment option for autoimmune diseases. Scientists believe that stem cells can help rebuild and repair damaged tissues in the body. This research is still in its early stages, but the potential benefits of stem cell therapy are exciting.

5. Nanotechnology

Nanotechnology holds immense promise for the future of autoimmune disease treatment. It involves using tiny particles to deliver medications to specific areas of the body. This type of targeted approach could decrease the need for large doses of medications and minimize side effects. In conclusion, there is a lot of potential for future treatments in the world of autoimmune disease research. Scientists are working tirelessly to better understand what causes these conditions and how to prevent or manage them effectively. With continued dedication to this field, there is hope that we will one day be able to cure these diseases once and for all.

SUBCHAPTER 6.2: POTENTIAL CURES FOR AUTOIMMUNE DISEASES

Despite the fact that autoimmune diseases are incurable, researchers continue to investigate possible treatment alternatives for these conditions. While there is no definitive cure for autoimmune diseases, there are several promising therapies that can alleviate symptoms and boost the quality of life of patients. Here are a few possible cures for autoimmune diseases:

1. Stem Cell Therapy:

Stem cell therapy is a method that has recently gained popularity in the medical community. This therapy entails transplanting healthy stem cells into the body to substitute infected or destroyed cells. When injected into the bloodstream, stem cells flock to the damaged area and differentiate into healthy cells, replacing the faulty cells that are causing the disease. Doctors have successfully used stem cell therapy to treat autoimmune diseases including Multiple Sclerosis, Crohn's Disease, and Psoriasis, as the stem cells can help regulate the immune system and reduce the severity of symptoms.

2. Immunotherapy:

Immunotherapy is a form of treatment that uses the immune system to fight illness. This type of therapy entails exposing the immune system to proteins, cells, and drugs that either direct the immune system to focus on the illness or to avoid destroying healthy tissues. Immunotherapy enables the immune system to effectively distinguish between invaders and healthy cells, reducing the severity of autoimmune conditions like rheumatoid arthritis and lupus.

3. Gene Editing:

Gene editing is another potential cure for certain autoimmune diseases. It entails modifying the genes that cause a specific illness to lower the occurrence of the disease symptoms. Researchers have made significant progress in gene-editing technology aimed at minimizing the flaws that cause autoimmune diseases such as type 1 diabetes and multiple sclerosis. Gene editing technology has the potential to cure autoimmune diseases, although it is still relatively new and requires more testing.

4. Biologic Therapies:

Biologic therapies are medications produced from living cells, bacteria, and viruses. This type of treatment targets the specific cells and proteins that contribute to the onset of autoimmune diseases. Biologic therapies act as immunomodulators, either dampening or stimulating the immune system depending on the context. These prescription medications are used to relieve symptoms and prevent disease advancement in autoimmune disorders such as rheumatoid arthritis, lupus, and psoriasis. In conclusion, while a definitive cure for autoimmune disease may be far off, substantial progress has been made in discovering and developing therapies that can relieve symptoms and prolong lives. Stem cell therapy, immunotherapy, gene editing, and biologic therapies hold the promise of long-awaited cures for autoimmune diseases. Researchers are also discovering the potential of diet and lifestyle changes in the management of these often-chronic diseases, giving hope to the millions of people living with autoimmune disorders every day.

COLLABORATIONS IN AUTOIMMUNE DISEASE RESEARCH

Collaboration is a fundamental aspect of advancing research on autoimmune diseases. With the complexity of these diseases, no single researcher or institution can achieve significant breakthroughs on their own. Collaborative research efforts promote the sharing of resources, knowledge, and expertise, leading to a deeper understanding of the underlying factors contributing to autoimmune diseases. One significant collaboration effort is the Autoimmunity Centers of Excellence (ACE) program, initiated by the National Institutes of Health (NIH). The program aims to bring together experts in various fields of basic, clinical, and translational research in autoimmune diseases to accelerate the pace of scientific breakthroughs. The ACE program encourages collaborations across institutions, disciplines, and government organizations to share resources, expertise, and technologies. Another collaboration effort is the Accelerating Medicines Partnership (AMP) program, a public-private partnership with the ambitious goal of speeding up the development of new treatments and diagnostics for autoimmune diseases. The program brings together leading scientists from academia, government, biotechnology, and pharmaceutical companies, collaborating on a wide range of tasks from analyzing big data to developing new technologies. Additionally, successful collaborations have led to the development of several inter-disciplinary research centers focused on autoimmune diseases, including the Harvard Medical School Immune Disease

Institute and the Johns Hopkins University Center for Autoimmune and Musculoskeletal Diseases. These centers provide a platform for bringing together experts in diverse fields such as immunology, genetics, microbiology, bioinformatics, and engineering to gain a deeper understanding of the complexities of autoimmune diseases and to develop innovative therapies. In conclusion, collaborations among researchers, institutions, and government organizations are crucial for advancing our understanding of autoimmune diseases. By pooling resources, knowledge, and expertise, researchers can accelerate scientific breakthroughs and develop innovative therapies for autoimmune diseases. The future of autoimmune disease research relies heavily on successful collaborations, and we can look forward to continued advances in our understanding and treatment of these complex diseases through these partnerships.

www.ingramcontent.com/pod-product-compliance
Lightning Source LLC
Chambersburg PA
CBHW051914250726
48659CB00002B/638